The Ultimate KETO Sweet Chaffle Recipe Book

Easy Sweet Chaffle Recipes For Beginners

Rory Kemp

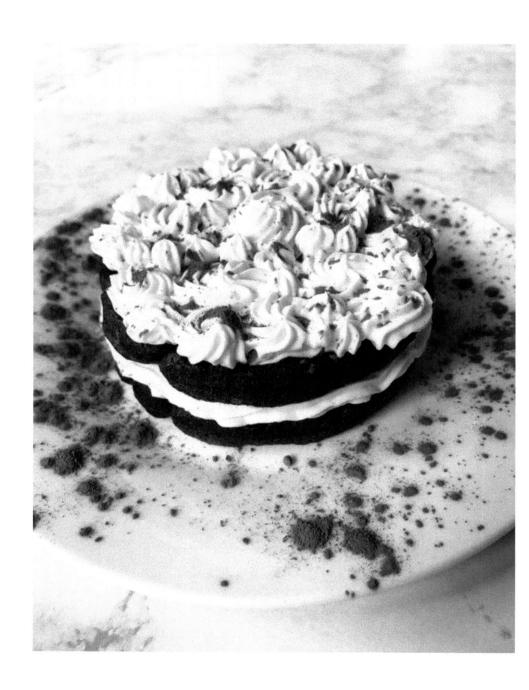

Table of contents

Chaffle Mascarpone and Cocoa..7

Blueberry Mousse Chaffle 9

Caramel & Chocolate Chips Chaffle 11

Vanilla & Coconut Whipped Cream Chaffle 13

Choco Coco Chaffle 15

Coconut Chaffle with Berries 17

Cereals & Walnuts Chaffle...19

Chocolate Chaffle with Eggnog Topping 21

Maple Syrup Crispy Chaffle.. 23

White Choco Lemon Chaffle 25

Cherry Chocolate Chaffle..27

Cherries Chaffle 29

Ricotta Lemon Chaffle..31

Pumpkin Cheesecake.. 33

Apples And Yogurt... 35

Keto Chaffle With Ice-cream...37

Chocolate Brownie Chaffles 39

Chaffle With Cream 41

Chocolate Chip Chaffle 43

Cinnamon Cream Cheese Chaffle 45

Christmas Smoothie with Chaffles 47

Raspberry And Chocolate Chaffle... 49

Almond Joy Cake Chaffle 51

Easy Maple Iced Soft Gingerbread Cookies Chaffle 54

Peanut Butter & Jelly Sammich Chaffle 56

Apple Pie Fries with Caramel Dipping Sauce 59

Apple Pie Churro Chaffle Tacos 63

Easy Soft Cinnamon Rolls Chaffle Cake 66

Mascarpone Cream Chaffle 67

Coffee Chaffle & Mascarpone Cream 69

Macadamia Nuts and Cinnamon Chaffle 71

Peppermint Chaffle 73

Berries Chaffle 75

Swiss Chocolate Chaffle 77

Chaffle Cereals 79

Whipped Cream Cereals Chaffle 81

Yogurt Green Chaffle 83

Almonds & Nutmeg Chaffle 85

Cashews Chaffle 87

Coconut Flakes Chaffle 89

Glazed Lemon Chaffle 91

Banana & Pecans Chaffle 93

Macadamia Nuts Chaffle 95

Peppermint and Choco Chips Chaffle 97

Almond Chocolate Chaffle and Jam 99

Caramel & Raspberries Chaffle 101

Choco & Coconut Whipped Cream Chaffle 103

Cereals & Raspberries Chaffle...105

Gourmet Eggnog Chaffle 107

Chaffle Mascarpone and Cocoa

Preparation: 5 minutes

Cooking: 8 minutes

Servings: 2 chaffles

Ingredients

For chaffles:

- 1 large egg, beaten
- ½ cup mozzarella cheese, shredded
- ½ tsp sweetener

For Mascarpone cream:

- 2 tbsp Mascarpone cheese, softened
- 2 tsp sweetener
- 1 tsp vanilla extract
- ½ tbsp unsalted butter, Melted
- ½ tbsp unsweetened cocoa powder

Directions

For mascarpone cream:

1. Add all the cream ingredients to a mixing bowl and Mix well until smoothy.

For Chaffle:

2. Heat up your waffle maker.
3. Add all the chaffles ingredients to a tiny mixing bowl and stir until well combined.
4. Pour half of the batter into your waffle maker and cook for 4 minutes until golden brown. Repeat now with the rest of the batter to make another chaffle.
5. Let cool for 3 minutes to let chaffles get crispy.
6. Serve with coconut flour and enjoy!

Blueberry Mousse Chaffle

Preparation: 5 minutes

Cooking: 8 minutes

Servings: 2 chaffles

Ingredients

For chaffles:

- 1 large egg, beaten
- ½ cup mozzarella cheese, grated
- 1 tsp coconut flour
- 1 tsp water
- ¼ tsp baking powder

For mousse:

- 2 tbsp heavy whipping cream
- 2-3 tbsp fresh blueberries
- ½ tsp lemon zest
- ½ tsp vanilla extract
- 1-2 fresh mint leaves, for garnish

Directions

For mousse:

1. In a bowl, whip all the mousse ingredients until fluffy. Set aside.

For chaffles:

1. Heat up the mini waffle maker.
2. Add all the chaffles ingredients to a tiny mixing bowl and combine well.
3. Pour half of the batter into your waffle maker and cook for 4 minutes until brown. Repeat now with the rest of the batter to make another chaffle.
4. Let cool for 3 minutes to let chaffles get crispy.
5. Top the chaffle with blueberry mousse and garnish with a fresh mint leaf.
6. Serve and enjoy!

Caramel & Chocolate Chips Chaffle

Preparation: 5 minutes

Cooking: 8 minutes

Servings: 2 chaffles

Ingredients

For chaffles:

- 1 egg, beaten
- ½ cup mozzarella cheese, grated
- 1 tsp coconut flour
- 1 tsp water
- ¼ tsp baking powder

For topping:

- 2 tbsp keto caramel sauce
- 2 tbsp chocolate chips, unsweetened
- 2 tsp sweetener

Directions

1. Heat up your waffle maker.

2. Add all the chaffles ingredients to a tiny mixing bowl and combine well.
3. Pour half of the batter into your waffle maker and cook for 4 minutes until brown. Repeat now with the rest of the batter to make another chaffle.
4. Let cool for 3 minutes to let chaffles get crispy.
5. Top the chaffles with caramel sauce and chocolate chips. Sprinkle with sweetener.
6. Serve and enjoy!

Vanilla & Coconut Whipped Cream Chaffle

Preparation: 5 minutes

Cooking: 8 minutes

Servings: 2 chaffles

Chaffles

- 1 tbsp almond flour
- ½ cup mozzarella cheese, shredded
- 1 egg, beaten
- 1 tbsp sweetener
- ½ teaspn vanilla extract
- 2 tbsp keto coconut whipped cream for topping

Directions

1. Heat up your waffle maker.
2. Add all the ingredients to a tiny mixing bowl and combine well.

3. Pour ½ of the batter into your waffle maker and cook for 4 minutes until golden brown. Cook the remaining batter to make another chaffle.
4. Top the chaffles with keto coconut whipped cream.
5. Serve and enjoy!

Choco Coco Chaffle

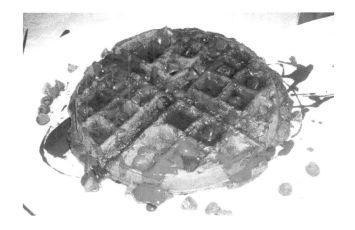

Preparation: 5 minutes

Cooking: 8 minutes

Servings: 2 chaffles

Ingredients

- 1 egg, beaten
- ½ cup mozzarella cheese, grated
- 1 tsp coconut flour
- 1 tsp water
- ¼ tsp baking powder
- 2 tbsp chocolate chips, unsweetened

Directions

1. Heat up your waffle maker.
2. Add all the ingredients to a tiny mixing bowl and stir until well combined.
3. Pour half of the batter into your waffle maker and cook for 4 minutes until brown. Repeat now with the rest of the batter to make another chaffle.
4. Let cool for 3 minutes to let chaffles get crispy.
5. Serve with cocoa powder and enjoy!

Coconut Chaffle with Berries

Preparation: 5 minutes

Cooking: 16 minutes

Servings: 4 chaffles

Ingredients

For chaffles:

- 2 tbsp softened cream cheese
- 2 eggs, beaten
- 1 cup mozzarella cheese, shredded
- 4 tbsp coconut flour
- 1 tsp baking powder
- 1 tbsp butter, Melted
- 2 tsp vanilla extract
- 1 tbsp sweetener

For topping:

- 4 tsp sweetener
- 4 tbsp fresh blackberries
- 4 tbsp fresh raspberries
- 4 tbsp fresh blueberries

Directions

1. Heat up your waffle maker.
2. Add all the chaffles ingredients to a tiny mixing bowl and stir until well combined.
3. Pour ¼ of the batter into your waffle maker and cook for 4 minutes. Then cook the remaining batter to make the other chaffles.
4. Top the chaffles with berries and sprinkle with sweetener.
5. Serve and enjoy!

Cereals & Walnuts Chaffle

Preparation: 5 minutes

Cooking: 8 minutes

Servings: 2 chaffles

Ingredients

- 1 large egg, beaten
- 2 tbsp almond flour
- 1 tbsp cereals, minced
- ¼ tsp baking powder
- 1 tbsp butter, Melted
- 1 tbsp cream cheese, softened
- ¼ tsp vanilla powder
- 1 tbsp sweetener
- ½ tbsp walnuts, chopped

Directions

1. Heat up your waffle maker.
2. Add all the ingredients to a tiny mixing bowl and stir until well combined.

3. Pour half of the batter into your waffle maker and cook for 4 minutes. Repeat now with the rest of the batter to make another chaffle.
4. Serve with keto caramel sauce and enjoy!

Chocolate Chaffle with Eggnog Topping

Preparation: 5 minutes

Cooking: 8 minutes

Servings: 2 chaffles

Ingredients

For chaffles:

- ½ cup shredded mozzarella cheese
- 1 tbsp almond flour
- 1 egg, beaten
- ¼ tsp cinnamon
- ½ tbsp sweetener
- 2 tbsp low carb chocolate chips

For topping:

- 2 tbsp Keto eggnog
- 2 tsp cinnamon powder

Directions

1. Heat up your waffle maker.

2. Add all the chaffles ingredients to a tiny mixing bowl and stir until well combined.
3. Add half of the batter into your waffle maker and cook it for approx. 4-5 minutes until golden brown. When the first one is completely done cooking, cook the second one.
4. Set aside for 1-2 minutes.
5. Top the chaffle with keto eggnog and sprinkle with cinnamon powder.
6. Serve and enjoy!

Maple Syrup Crispy Chaffle

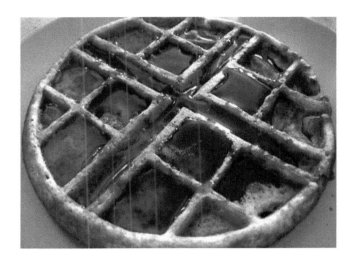

Preparation: 5 minutes

Cooking: 8 minutes

Servings: 2 chaffles

Ingredients

- 1 large egg, beaten
- ¼ cup parmesan cheese, shredded
- ½ cup mozzarella cheese, shredded
- 2 tbsp unsweetened maple syrup for topping

Directions

1. Heat up your waffle maker.
2. Add all the chaffles ingredients except for parmesan cheese to a tiny mixing bowl and combine well.
3. Pour half of the batter into your waffle maker, sprinkle with 1-2 tbsp of shredded parmesan cheese and cook for 4 minutes until golden brown. Repeat now with the rest of the batter to make another chaffle.
4. Let cool for 3 minutes to let chaffles get crispy.
5. Top the chaffles with keto maple syrup.
6. Serve with coconut flour and enjoy!

White Choco Lemon Chaffle

Preparation: 5 minutes

Cooking: 8 minutes

Servings: 2 chaffles

Ingredients

For chaffles:

- 1 large egg, beaten
- ½ tbsp butter, Melted
- ½ tbsp softened cream cheese
- 1 tbsp unsweetened white chocolate chips
- 1 tbsp almond flour
- 1 tsp coconut flour
- 1 tbsp sweetener
- ¼ tsp baking powder
- ¼ tsp vanilla extract

Ingredients for lemon icing:

- 2 tbsp sweetener
- 4 tsp heavy cream
- 1 tsp lemon juice

25

- Fresh lemon zest

Directions

1. Heat up your waffle maker.
2. Add all the chaffles ingredients to a tiny mixing bowl and stir until well combined.
3. Pour half of the batter into your waffle maker and cook for 4 minutes. Repeat now with the rest of the batter to prepare the other chaffle.
4. Let cool for 3 minutes to let chaffles get crispy.
5. Combine in a mixing bowl the sweetener, heavy cream, lemon juice and lemon zest. Pour over the chaffles.
6. Serve and enjoy!

Cherry Chocolate Chaffle

Preparation: 15 minutes

Cooking: 10 Minutes

Servings: 1

Ingredients

- 1 egg, lightly beaten
- 1 tbsp. unsweetened chocolate chips
- 2 tbsp. sugar-free cherry pie filling
- 2 tbsp. heavy whipping cream
- 1/2 cup Mozzarella cheese, shredded
- 1/2 tsp. baking powder, gluten-free
- 1 tbsp. Swerve
- 1 tbsp. unsweetened cocoa powder
- 1 tbsp. almond flour

Directions

1. Preheat now your waffle maker.
2. In a bowl, whisk together egg, cheese, baking powder, Swerve, cocoa powder, and almond flour.

3. Spray waffle maker with cooking spray.
4. Pour batter in the hot waffle maker and cooking until golden brown.
5. Top with cherry pie filling, heavy whipping cream, and chocolate chips and serve.

Nutrition

Kcal 468, Fat 39.5g, Net Carbs 2g, Protein 26g:

Cherries Chaffle

Preparation: 5 minutes

Cooking: 8 minutes

Servings: 2 chaffles

Ingredients

For chaffles:

- 1 large egg, beaten
- ½ cup mozzarella cheese, shredded
- ¼ tsp sweetener

For topping:

- 2 tbsp dark sweet cherries, halved
- 2 tbsp keto whipped heavy cream
- 2 tsp sweetener

Directions

1. Heat up your waffle maker.
2. Add all the chaffles ingredients to a tiny mixing bowl and stir until well combined.

3. Pour half of the batter into your waffle maker and cook for 4 min, until brown. Repeat now with the rest of the batter to make another chaffle.
4. Let cool for 3 minutes to let chaffles get crispy.
5. Spread the chaffles with whipped heavy cream, add cherries and sprinkle with sweetener.
6. Serve and enjoy!

Ricotta Lemon Chaffle

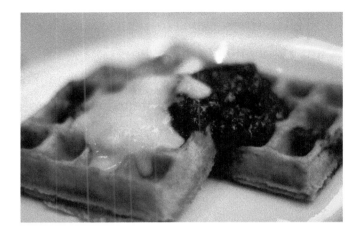

Preparation: 5 minutes

Cooking: 8 minutes

Servings: 2 chaffles

Ingredients

- 1 large egg, beaten
- ½ cup skim ricotta cheese
- 1 tbsp almond flour
- ½ tsp baking powder
- ½ tsp fresh lemon zest
- ½ tsp fresh lemon juice

Directions

1. Heat up your waffle maker.
2. Add all the ingredients to a tiny mixing bowl and stir until well combined.
3. Pour half of the batter into your waffle maker and cook for 4 minutes until golden brown. Repeat now with the rest of the batter to make another chaffle.
4. Let cool for 3 minutes to let chaffles get crispy.
5. Serve and enjoy!

Pumpkin Cheesecake

Cooking: 15 Minutes

Servings: 2

Ingredients

<u>For chaffle:</u>

- 1 egg
- 1/2 tsp vanilla
- 1/2 tsp baking powder, gluten-free
- 1/4 tsp pumpkin spice
- 1 tsp cream cheese, softened
- 2 tsp heavy cream
- 1 tbsp Swerve
- 1 tbsp almond flour
- 2 tsp pumpkin puree
- 1/2 cup mozzarella cheese, shredded

<u>For filling:</u>

- 1/4 tsp vanilla
- 1 tbsp Swerve
- 2 tbsp cream cheese

Directions:

1. Preheat now your mini waffle maker.
2. In a tiny bowl, mix all chaffle Ingredients.
3. Spray waffle maker with cooking spray.
4. Pour half batter in the hot waffle maker and cook for 3-5 minutes. Repeat now with the remaining batter.
5. In a tiny bowl, combine all filling Ingredients.
6. Spread Ming mixture between two chaffles and place in the fridge for 10 minutes.
7. Serve and enjoy.

Nutrition:

Calories 107, Fat 7.2 g, Carbohydrates 5 g, Sugar 0.7 mg, Sodium 207 mg, Potassium 15mg, Total Carbohydrate 1 g, Dietary Fiber 1 g, Protein 10 g, Total Sugars 1 g ,

Apples And Yogurt

Cooking: 10 Minutes

Servings: 2

Ingredients

- 1 tbspn unsalted butter
- 1 tbspn golden brown sugar
- 1 Granny Smith apple, cored and thinly sliced
- 1 pinch salt
- 2 whole-grain frozen waffles, toasted
- 1/2 cup mozzarella cheese, shredded
- 1/4 cup Yoplait® Original French
- Vanilla yogurt

Directions

1. Melt now the butter in a large skillet over medium-high heat until brown. Add mozzarella cheese and stir well.
2. Add the sugar, apple slices, salt, and cook, stirring frequently until apples are softened and tender, about 6 to 9 minutes.

3. Put one warm waffle each on a plate, top each with yogurt and apples. Serve warm.

Nutrition:

Calories: 240, Total Fat: 10.4 g, Cholesterol: 54 mg, Sodium: 226 mg, Total Carbohydrate: 33.8 g, Protein: 4.7 g

Keto Chaffle With Ice-cream

Cooking: 5 Minutes

Servings: 2

Ingredients

- 1 egg
- 1/2 cup cheddar cheese, shredded
- 1 tbsp. almond flour
- 1/2 tsp. baking powder.

For Serving:

- 1/2 cup heavy cream
- 1 tbsp. keto chocolate chips.
- 2 oz. raspberries
- 2 oz. blueberries

Directions:

1. Preheat now your waffle maker according to the manufacturer's Directions
2. Mix chaffle ingredients in a tiny bowl and make chaffles.
3. For an ice-cream ball, mix cream and chocolate chips in a bowl and pour this mixture in 2 silicone molds.

4. Freeze the ice-cream balls in a freezer for about 2-hours.
5. For serving, set ice-cream ball on chaffle.
6. Top with berries and enjoy!

Nutrition:

Protein: 147 kcal, Fat: 80% 219 kcal, Carbohydrates: 3% 7 kcal

Chocolate Brownie Chaffles

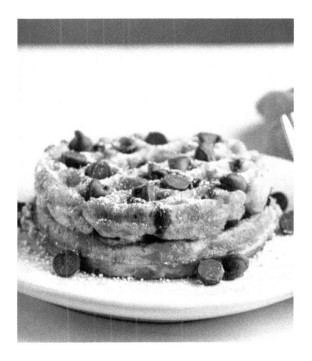

Cooking: 5 minutes

Servings: 2

Ingredients

- 2 tbsp. cocoa powder
- 1 egg
- 1/4 tsp baking powder
- 1 tbsp. heavy whipping cream

- 1/2 cup mozzarella cheese

Directions

1. Beat egg with a fork in a tiny mixing bowl.
2. Add the remaining ingredients in a beaten egg and beat well with a beater until the mixture is smooth and fluffy.
3. Pour batter in a greased Preheat nowed waffle maker.
4. Close the lid.
5. Cook chaffles for about 4 minutes until they are thoroughly cooked.
6. Serve with berries and enjoy!

Nutrition:

Protein: 32% 51 kcal, Fat: 62% 100 kcal, Carbohydrates: 6% 10 kcal

Chaffle With Cream

Cooking: 5 minutes

Servings: 4

Ingredients

- 1 cup egg whites
- 1/2 tsp. of vanilla
- 1 tsp. baking powder
- 1 cup mozzarella cheese, grated

Topping:

- 1/2 cup frozen heavy cream
- Cherries

Directions

1. Switch on your square waffle maker. Spray with non-stick spray.
2. Beat egg whites with beater, until fluffy and white.
3. Stir in the cheese, baking powder and vanilla.
4. Pour 1/2 of the batter in a waffle maker.
5. Close the maker and cook for about 3 minutes.
6. Repeat now with the remaining batter.
7. Remove now chaffles from the maker.

8. Serve with heavy cream and cherries on top and enjoy!

Nutrition:

Protein: 38% 133 kcal, Fat: 57% 201 kcal Carbohydrates: 5% 18 kcal

Chocolate Chip Chaffle

Cooking: 8 Minutes

Servings: 2

Ingredients

- 1 egg
- 1/2 teaspn coconut flour
- 1/4 teaspn baking powder
- 1 teaspn sweetener
- 1 tbspn heavy whipping cream
- 1 tbspn chocolate chips

Directions

1. Preheat now your waffle maker.
2. Beat the egg in a bowl.
3. Stir in the flour, baking powder, sweetener and cream.
4. Pour half of the mixture into your waffle maker.
5. Sprinkle the chocolate chips on top and close.
6. Cook for 4 minutes.
7. Remove now the chaffle and put on a plate.

8. Do the same procedure with the remaining batter.

Nutrition:

Calories 146, Total Fat 10 g, Saturated Fat 7 g, Cholesterol 88 mg, Sodium 140 mg, Potassium 50 mg, Total Carbohydrate 5 g, Dietary Fiber 3 g, Protein 6 g, Total Sugars 1 g

Cinnamon Cream Cheese Chaffle

Cooking: 15 Minutes

Servings: 2

Ingredients

- 2 eggs, lightly beaten
- 1 tsp collagen
- 1/4 tsp baking powder, gluten-free
- 1 tsp monk fruit sweetener
- 1/2 tsp cinnamon
- 1/4 cup cream cheese, softened
- Pinch of salt

Directions

1. Preheat now your waffle maker.
2. Add all ingredients into the bowl and beat using hand mixer until well combined.
3. Spray waffle maker with cooking spray.
4. Pour 1/2 batter in the hot waffle maker and cook for 3-minutes or until golden brown. Repeat now with the remaining batter.
5. Serve and enjoy.

Nutrition:

Calories 179, Fat 14.5 g, Carbohydrates 1.9 g, Sugar 0.4 g, Protein 10.8 g, Cholesterol 19mg

Christmas Smoothie with Chaffles

Cooking: 10 Minutes

Servings: 2

Ingredients

- 1 cup coconut milk
- 2 tbsps. almonds chopped
- 1/4 cup cherries
- 1 pinch sea salt
- 1/4 cup ice cubes

For Topping:

- 2 oz. keto chocolate chips
- 2 oz. cherries
- 2 scoop heavy cream, frozen

Directions

1. Add almond milk, almonds, cherries, salt and ice in a blender, blend for 2 minutes until smooth and fluffy.
2. Pour the smoothie into glasses.
3. Top with one scoop heavy cream, chocolate chips, cherries and chaffle in each glass.

4. Serve and enjoy!

Nutrition:

Protein: 4% 11 kcal, Fat: 84% 24 kcal, Carbohydrates: 13% 37 kcal

Raspberry And Chocolate Chaffle

Cooking: 7-9 Minutes

Servings: 4

Ingredients

Batter:

- 4 eggs
- 2 ounce ofs cream cheese, softened
- 2 ounce ofs sour cream
- 1 teaspn vanilla extract
- 5 tbsps almond flour
- 1/4 cup cocoa powder
- 1.1/2 teaspns baking powder
- 2 ounce ofs fresh or frozen raspberries

Other:

- 2 tbsps butter to brush your waffle maker
- Fresh sprigs of mint to garnish

Directions

1. Preheat now your waffle maker.

2. Add the eggs, cream cheese and sour cream to a bowl and stir with a wire whisk until combined.
3. Add the vanilla extract and Mix well until combined.
4. Stir in the almond flour, cocoa powder, and baking powder and Mix well until combined.
5. Add the raspberries and stir until combined.
6. Brush the heated waffle maker with butter and add a few tbsps of the batter.
7. Close the lid and cook for about 8 minutes depending on your waffle maker.
8. Serve with fresh sprigs of mint.

Nutrition:

Calories 270, Fat 23 g, Carbs 8.g, Sugar 1.3 g, Protein 10.2 g, Sodium 158 mg

Almond Joy Cake Chaffle

Preparation: 18-20 minutes

Servings: 6

Ingredients

Chocolate Chaffles:

- 1 egg
- 1 ounce of cream cheese
- 1 tbspn almond flour
- 1 tbspn unsweetened cocoa powder
- 1 tbspn erythritol sweetener blend such as Swerve, Pyure or Lakanto
- 1/2 teaspn vanilla extract
- 1/4 teaspn instant coffee powder

Coconut Filling:

- 1.1/2 teaspns coconut oil Melted
- 1 tbspn heavy cream
- 1/4 cup unsweetened finely shredded coconut
- 2 ounce ofs cream cheese
- 1 tbspn confectioner's sweetener such as Swerve
- 1/4 teaspn vanilla extract

- 14 whole almonds

Directions

For the Chaffles:

1. Preheat now your waffle iron until thoroughly hot.
2. In a bowl, whisk all chaffle ingredients together until well combined.
3. Pour half of the batter into waffle iron.
4. Close and cook 3-5 min, until done. Remove now to a wire rack.
5. Repeat for the second chaffle.

For the Filing:

6. Soften cream to room temperature or warm in the microwave for 10 seconds.
7. Add all ingredients to a bowl and mix well until smooth and well-combined.

Assembly:

8. Spread half the filling on one chaffle and place 7 almonds evenly on top of the filling.
9. Repeat now with the second chaffle and stack together.

Nutrition:

Calories: 130kcal, Carbohydrates: 6.3g, Protein: 3g, Fat: 10.6g, Fiber: 1g, Sugar: 3.4g

Easy Maple Iced Soft Gingerbread Cookies Chaffle

Preparation: 20 minutes

Servings: 2

Ingredients

Chaffles:

- 1 egg
- 1 ounce of cream cheese softened to room temperature
- 2 teaspns Melted butter
- 1 tbspn Swerve Brown sweetener
- 1 tbspn almond flour
- 2 teaspns coconut flour
- 1/4 teaspn baking powder
- 3/4 teaspn ground ginger
- 1/2 teaspn ground cinnamon
- Generous dash ground nutmeg
- Generous dash ground clove

<u>Icing:</u>

- 2 tbsps powdered sweeteners such as Swerve or Lakanto
- 1 1/2 teaspns heavy cream
- 1/8 teaspn maple extract
- Water as needed to thin the frosting

Directions

1. Heat waffle iron until thoroughly hot.
2. Beat all chaffle ingredients together in a tiny bowl until smooth.
3. Add a heaping 2 tbsps of batter to waffle iron and cook until done about 4 minutes.
4. Repeat to make 2 chaffles. Let cool on wire rack.

<u>Maple Icing</u>**:**

5. In a tiny bowl whisk together sweetener, heavy cream, and maple extract until smooth.
6. Add enough water to thin to a spreadable consistency. (I used about 1 teaspn water.)
7. Spread icing on each chaffle and sprinkle with additional ground cinnamon, if desired

Peanut Butter & Jelly Sammich Chaffle

Preparation: 20 minutes

Cooking: 30 minutes

Servings: 2

Ingredients

For Chaffle:

- Egg: 2
- Mozzarella: ¼ cup
- Vanilla extract: 1 tbsp.
- Coconut flour: 2 tbsp.
- Baking powder: ¼ tsp.
- Cinnamon powder: 1 tsp.
- Swerve sweetener: 1 tbsp.

For Blueberry Compote:

- Blueberries: 1 cup
- Lemon zest: ½ tsp.
- Lemon juice: 1 tsp.
- Xanthan gum: 1/8 tsp.
- Water: 2 tbsp.

- Swerve sweetener: 1 tbsp.

Directions

1. For the blueberry compote, add all the ingredients except xanthan gum to a tiny pan
2. Mix now them all and boil
3. Lower the heat and simmer for 8-10 minutes; the sauce will initiate to thicken
4. Add xanthan gum now and stir
5. Now Remove now the pan from the stove and allow the mixture to cool down
6. Put in refrigerator
7. Preheat now a mini waffle maker if needed and grease it
8. In a mixing bowl, add all the chaffle ingredients and mix well
9. Pour the mixture to the lower plate of your waffle maker and spread it evenly to cover the plate properly
10. Close the lid
11. Cooking for at least 4 minutes to get the desired crunch
12. Remove now the chaffle from the heat and keep aside

13. Make as many chaffles as your mixture and waffle maker allow

14. Serve with the blueberry and enjoy!

Nutrition:

Calories: 175; Total Fat: 15g; Carbs: 8g; Net Carbs: 5g; Fiber: 3g; Protein: 6g

Apple Pie Fries with Caramel Dipping Sauce

Preparation: 30-35 minutes

Servings: 2

Ingredients

(Egg-Free) Fathead Pie Dough:

- 1 cup mozzarella whole milk, shredded
- 1/2 cup almond flour superfine
- 1/2 T Swerve Confectioners
- 1 T cream cheese full fat
- 1/4 tsp glucomannan helps dough crisp

Jicama "Apple" Pie Filling:

- 1 cup jicama chopped tiny
- 2 T Swerve Brown
- 2 T butter
- 1/2 T apple pie spice
- 1/2 tsp apple extract
- 1/4 tsp vanilla extract
- 1 packet True Lemon

Cinnamon Sugar:

- 2 T Swerve Brown
- 1/2 tsp Ceylon Cinnamon

Caramel Dipping Sauce:

- 2 T butter
- 2 T Swerve Brown
- 1 T Swerve Confectioners
- 1/4 cup heavy cream
- 1/8 tsp xanthan gum
- 1/8 tsp kosher or sea salt
- 1 tbsp water

Directions

(Egg-Free) Fathead Pie Dough:

1. Place the mozzarella and cream cheese in a microwaveable bowl.
2. Microwave for 1 minute, stir and then cook for another 30 seconds.
3. Stir in sweetener, almond flour, and glucomannan.
4. Let the dough cool slightly, then knead until smooth.
5. Roll out dough between two pieces of parchment paper. The thinner you roll the dough the crispier your "fries" will be.

6. Cut out circles with 3-4 inch cookie cutter.
7. Take scraps and knead together. You may need to reheat slightly.
8. Continue cutting circles until all dough is used.

Jicama "Apple" Pie Filling:

9. Combine chopped jicama with butter, sweetener, lemon packet and spices in a pan.
10. Cook and stir over medium heat until jicama has softened.
11. Remove now from heat and add apple and vanilla extracts.
12. Let cool slightly before adding to a food processor. Pulse until filling is smooth.

Cinnamon Sugar:

1. Preheat now the GRIDDLE.
2. Place one dough circle on the grill.
3. Add 1-2 tsp of "apple" filling and top with another piece of dough.
4. Cook 3-4 minutes until golden.
5. Sprinkle with Cinnamon Sugar mixture generously on both sides of the pie immediately after removing from the dash griddle.
6. Place on a cooling rack.
7. When fully cooled (put in the fridge to speed up cooling) slice into fries!

8. Dip in your favorite caramel sauce or whipped cream and enjoy!

Caramel Dipping Sauce:

1. Combine butter and sweeteners in a tiny saucepan.
2. Bring to a boil over medium heat and cook 3 to 5 minutes(careful not to burn it).
3. Remove now from heat and add cream. The mixture will bubble vigorously.
4. Sprinkle with xanthan gum and whisk to combine.
5. Add salt.
6. Return mixture to heat and boil 1 more minute.
7. Let cool to lukewarm and stir in water until well combined.

Apple Pie Churro Chaffle Tacos

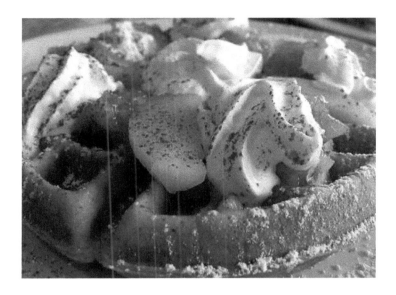

Preparation: 1 hour

Servings: 2

Ingredients

<u>Chayote Apple Pie Filling</u>

- 1 Chayote Squash cooked, peeled and sliced
- 1 T Kerrygold butter Melted
- 2 packets True Lemon
- 1/8 tsp cream of tartar
- 1/4 cup Swerve Brown

- 2 tsp Ceylon cinnamon powder more if you like
- 1/8 tsp ginger powder
- 1/8 tsp nutmeg

Cinnamon Chaffle:

- 2 eggs room temperature
- 1/4 cup mozzarella shredded
- 1 tsp Ceylon cinnamon
- 1 T Swerve Confectioners
- 2 tsp coconut flour
- 1/8 tsp baking powder
- 1 tsp vanilla extract

Directions

Apple Pie Taco Filling:

1. Boil the whole chayote for 25 minutes. Let it cool. Peel and slice into 1/4 inch slices.
2. Mix all ingredients together and stir in chayote to coat well.
3. Place in a tiny baking dish and cover with foil. Bake for 20 minutes.
4. Place 1/4 of the mixture in a food processor or tiny blender and process until it reaches applesauce consistency.

5. Add to chayote slices and stir.

Apple Pie Churro Chaffle Taco:

6. Whip eggs.
7. Add sweetener, cinnamon, and vanilla.
8. Mix well.
9. Add remaining ingredients and stir.
10. Put 3 T batter in Preheated Griddle.
11. Cook for 5 minutes.
12. Sprinkle hot chaffle with cinnamon and granular sweetener mixture.

To Assemble:

13. Place chaffles in taco holders or fold gently to shape.
14. Add 1/4 of Apple filling to each taco chaffle.
15. Top with whipped cream or vanilla bean ice cream.

Easy Soft Cinnamon Rolls Chaffle Cake

Preparation: 15 minutes

Servings: 2

Ingredients

- 1 egg
- 1/2 cup mozzarella cheese
- 1/2 tsp vanilla
- 1/2 tsp cinnamon
- 1 tbs monk fruit confectioners blend

Directions

1. Preheat now waffle maker.
2. In a tiny bowl, whip the egg.
3. Add the remaining Ingredients.
4. Spray your waffle maker with non-stick cooking spray.
5. Makes 2 chaffles.
6. Divide mixture.
7. Cook half the mixture for about 4 minutes or until golden brown.

Mascarpone Cream Chaffle

Preparation: 5 minutes

Cooking: 8 minutes

Servings: 2 chaffles

Ingredients

For chaffles:

- 1 large egg, beaten
- ½ cup mozzarella cheese, shredded
- ½ tsp sweetener

For Mascarpone cream:

- 2 tbsp Mascarpone cheese, softened
- 2 tsp sweetener
- 1 tsp vanilla extract
- ½ tbsp unsalted butter, Melted
- 2 tsp unsweetened cocoa powder for topping

Directions

For mascarpone cream:

1. Add all the cream ingredients to a mixing bowl and Mix well until smoothy.

For Chaffle:

2. Heat up your waffle maker.
3. Add all the chaffles ingredients to a tiny mixing bowl and stir until well combined.
4. Pour half of the batter into your waffle maker and cook for 4 minutes until golden brown. Repeat now with the rest of the batter to make another chaffle.
5. Let cool for 3 minutes to let chaffles get crispy.
6. Spread the chaffles with mascarpone cream and sprinkle with cocoa powder.
7. Serve and enjoy!

Coffee Chaffle & Mascarpone Cream

Preparation: 5 minutes

Cooking: 8 minutes

Servings: 2 chaffles

Ingredients

For chaffles:

- 1 large egg, beaten
- 1 tsp sweetener
- ¼ tsp baking powder
- ½ cup softened cream cheese
- ¼ tsp instant coffee powder

Ingredients for Mascarpone cream:

- 2 tbsp Mascarpone cheese, softened
- 2 tsp sweetener
- 1 tsp vanilla extract
- ½ tbsp unsalted butter, Melted

Directions

For mascarpone cream:

1. Add all the cream ingredients to a mixing bowl and Mix well until smoothy.

For chaffles:

2. Heat up your waffle maker.
3. Add all the chaffles ingredients to a tiny mixing bowl and stir until well combined.
4. Pour half of the batter into your waffle maker and cook for 4 minutes until golden brown. Repeat now with the rest of the batter to make another chaffle.
5. Let cool for 3 minutes to let chaffles get crispy.
6. Spread the chaffle with mascarpone cream.
7. Serve and enjoy!

Macadamia Nuts and Cinnamon Chaffle

Preparation: 5 minutes

Cooking: 8 minutes

Servings: 2 chaffles

Ingredients

For chaffles:

- 1 tbsp almond flour
- ½ cup mozzarella cheese, shredded
- 1 egg, beaten
- 1 tbsp sweetener
- ½ tsp vanilla extract
- A pinch of salt
- 1 tbsp Macadamia nuts, minced
- ½ tsp cinnamon powder

Directions

1. Heat up your waffle maker.
2. Add all the ingredients to a tiny mixing bowl and combine well.

3. Pour ½ of the batter into your waffle maker and cook for 4 minutes until golden brown. Then cook the remaining batter to make another chaffle.
4. Top the chaffles with unsweetened maple syrup.
5. Serve and enjoy!

Peppermint Chaffle

Preparation: 5 minutes

Cooking: 8 minutes

Servings: 2 chaffles

Ingredients

- 1 tbsp almond flour
- ½ cup mozzarella cheese, shredded
- 1 egg, beaten
- 1 tbsp sweetener
- ½ tsp vanilla extract
- 3-4 chopped mint leaves
- A pinch of salt

Directions

1. Heat up your waffle maker.
2. Add all the ingredients to a tiny mixing bowl and combine well.

3. Pour ½ of the batter into your waffle maker and cook for 4 minutes until golden brown. Then cook the remaining batter to make another chaffle.
4. Top the chaffles with keto ice cream.
5. Serve and enjoy!

Berries Chaffle

Preparation: 5 minutes

Cooking: 16 minutes

Servings: 4 chaffles

Ingredients

- 1 cup of mozzarella cheese, shredded
- 2 tbsp almond flour
- 2 tsp of sweetener
- ½ tbsp blackberries
- ½ tbsp cranberries
- 1 tsp baking powder
- 2 eggs, beaten
- 1 tsp cinnamon
- 2 tbsp heavy cream for the topping

Directions

1. Heat up your waffle maker.

2. Add the mozzarella cheese, baking powder, almond flour, eggs, cinnamon, sweetener, and berries to a medium mixing bowl. Mix well.
3. Spray your waffle maker with a cooking spray.
4. Add in about ¼ a cup of batter. Cook the chaffle for 4-5 minutes until it is crispy and brown. Repeat now with the remaining batter to prepare the other chaffles.
5. Serve with heavy cream and enjoy!

Swiss Chocolate Chaffle

Preparation: 5 minutes

Cooking: 8 minutes

Servings: 2 chaffles

Ingredients

- 1 egg, beaten
- ½ cup mozzarella cheese, shredded
- 1 tbsp cream cheese
- 1 tbsp sweetener
- 2 tsp coconut flour
- ¼ tsp baking powder
- 1 tbsp unsweetened cocoa powder
- 1 tbsp unsweetened chocolate chips

Directions

1. Heat up your waffle maker.
2. Add all the ingredients to a tiny mixing bowl and stir until well combined.

3. Pour half of the batter into your waffle maker and cook for 4 minutes until golden brown. Repeat now with the rest of the batter to make another chaffle.
4. Serve and enjoy!

Chaffle Cereals

Preparation: 5 minutes

Cooking: 8 minutes

Servings: 2 chaffles

Ingredients

- 1 large egg, beaten
- ½ cup mozzarella cheese, shredded
- 2 tbsp almond flour
- ½ tsp coconut flour
- 1 tbsp cereals, minced
- ¼ tsp baking powder
- 1 tbsp butter, Melted
- 1 tbsp cream cheese
- ¼ tsp vanilla powder
- 1 tbsp sweetener

Directions

1. Heat up your waffle maker.

2. Add all the ingredients to a tiny mixing bowl and stir until well combined.

3. Pour half of the batter into your waffle maker and cook for 4 minutes. Repeat now with the rest of the batter to make another chaffle.

4. Serve and enjoy!

Whipped Cream Cereals Chaffle

Preparation: 5 minutes

Cooking: 8 minutes

Servings: 2 chaffles

Ingredients

- 1 large egg, beaten
- ½ cup mozzarella cheese, shredded
- 2 tbsp almond flour
- ½ tsp coconut flour
- 1 tbsp cereals, minced
- ¼ tsp baking powder
- 1 tbsp butter, Melted
- 1 tbsp cream cheese
- ¼ tsp vanilla powder
- 1 tbsp sweetener

For topping:

- 2 tbsp whipped cream, unsweetened
- 2 tsp maple syrup, unsweetened

Directions

1. Heat up your waffle maker.
2. Add all the chaffles ingredients to a tiny mixing bowl and stir until well combined.
3. Pour half of the batter into your waffle maker and cook for 4 minutes. Repeat now with the rest of the batter to make another chaffle.
4. Top the chaffles with whipped cream and maple syrup.
5. Serve and enjoy!

Yogurt Green Chaffle

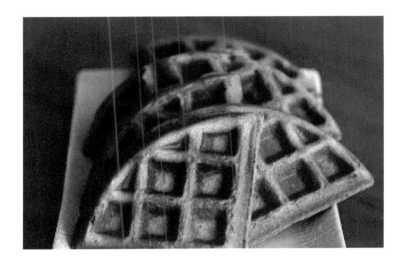

Preparation: 5 minutes

Cooking: 8 minutes

Servings: 2 chaffles

Ingredients

- ½ tsp psyllium husk
- ½ cup mozzarella cheese, shredded
- 1 egg, beaten
- 1 tbsp yogurt
- ¼ tsp baking powder

- 1 tiny avocado, sliced for topping

Directions

1. Heat up the mini waffle maker.
2. Add all the ingredients to a tiny mixing bowl and stir until well combined.
3. Pour half of the batter into your waffle maker and cook for 4 minutes until brown. Repeat now with the rest of the batter to prepare another chaffle.
4. Top the chaffles with sliced avocado.
5. Serve and enjoy!

Almonds & Nutmeg Chaffle

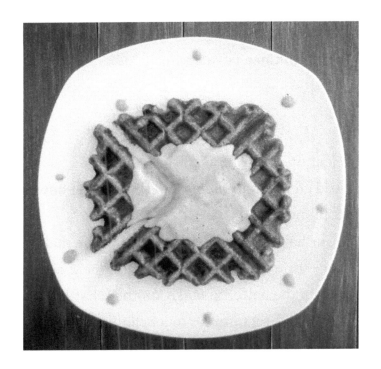

Preparation: 5 minutes

Cooking: 8 minutes

Servings: 2 chaffles

Ingredients

- 1 large egg, beaten
- ½ cup of mozzarella cheese, shredded

- 2 tbsp almond flour
- ¼ tsp baking powder
- 2 tbsp almonds, chopped
- ¼ tsp nutmeg powder

Directions

1. Heat up your waffle maker.
2. Add all the ingredients to a tiny mixing bowl and combine well.
3. Pour half of the batter into your waffle maker and cook for 4 minutes until brown. Repeat now with the rest of the batter to make another chaffle.
4. Let cool for 3 minutes to let chaffles get crispy.
5. Serve with keto whipped cream and enjoy!

Cashews Chaffle

Preparation: 5 minutes

Cooking: 8 minutes

Servings: 2 chaffles

Ingredients

- 1 egg, beaten
- ½ cup mozzarella cheese, grated
- 1 tsp coconut flour
- 1 tsp water
- ¼ tsp baking powder
- 2 tbsp cashews, chopped for topping

Directions

1. Heat up the mini waffle maker.
2. Add all the ingredients to a tiny mixing bowl and combine well.
3. Pour half of the batter into your waffle maker and cook for 4 minutes until brown. Repeat now with the rest of the batter to make another chaffle.

4. Let cool for 3 minutes to let chaffles get crispy.
5. Garnish with chopped cashews and unsweetened maple syrup.
6. Serve and enjoy!

Coconut Flakes Chaffle

Preparation: 5 minutes

Cooking: 8 minutes

Servings: 2 chaffles

Ingredients

For chaffles:

- 1 egg, beaten
- ½ cup mozzarella cheese, grated
- 1 tsp coconut flour
- 1 tsp water
- ¼ tsp baking powder

For topping:

- 2 tbsp caramel sauce, unsweetened
- 2 tbsp coconut flakes

Directions

1. Heat up the mini waffle maker.
2. Add all the chaffles ingredients to a tiny mixing bowl and combine well.

3. Pour half of the batter into your waffle maker and cook for 4 minutes until brown. Repeat now with the rest of the batter to make another chaffle.
4. Let cool for 3 minutes to let chaffles get crispy.
5. Top the chaffles with caramel sauce and coconut flakes.
6. Serve and enjoy!

Glazed Lemon Chaffle

Preparation: 9 minutes

Cooking: 4 minutes

Servings: 1 chaffle

Ingredients

For chaffles:

- 1 tbsp heavy whipping cream
- 1 tbsp sweetener
- 1 tbsp coconut flour
- 1 egg
- ½ cup mozzarella cheese, shredded
- ½ tsp lemon extract
- ¼ tsp lemon zest

For the glaze:

- 2 tsp lemon Juice
- 2 tbsp sweetener

Directions

1. Heat up your waffle maker.

2. Mix all the ingredients in a tiny mixing bowl and blend until creamy.
3. Pour the batter into your waffle maker and cook for about 4 minutes.
4. Whisk the lemon juice and the sweetener for the glaze in a mixing bowl, adding lemon juice until your desired consistency has been reached.
5. Pour the glaze over the chaffle.
6. Serve and enjoy!

Banana & Pecans Chaffle

Preparation: 5 minutes

Cooking: 8 minutes

Servings: 2 chaffles

Ingredients

- 1 tbsp cream cheese
- 1 tbsp sweetener
- 1 egg
- ½ cup of mozzarella cheese, shredded
- ½ tsp vanilla extract
- 1 tsp banana extract, sugar-free
- 1 tbsp pecans, chopped for topping

Directions

1. Heat up the mini waffle maker.
2. Add all the ingredients to a tiny mixing bowl and stir until well combined.
3. Pour half of the batter into your waffle maker and cook for 4 minutes until brown.

4. Repeat now with the remaining batter to prepare another chaffle.
5. Let cool for 3 minutes to let chaffles get crispy.
6. Serve and enjoy!

Macadamia Nuts Chaffle

Preparation: 5 minutes

Cooking: 8 minutes

Servings: 2 chaffles

Ingredients

- 1 tbsp almond flour
- ½ cup mozzarella cheese, shredded
- 1 egg, beaten
- 1 tbsp sweetener
- ½ tsp vanilla extract
- A pinch of salt
- 1 tbsp Macadamia nuts, minced

Directions

1. Heat up your waffle maker.
2. Add all the ingredients to a tiny mixing bowl and combine well.

3. Pour ½ of the batter into your waffle maker and cook for 4 minutes until golden brown. Then cook the remaining batter to make another chaffle.
4. Top the chaffles with keto whipped cream.
5. Serve and enjoy!

Peppermint and Choco Chips Chaffle

Preparation: 5 minutes

Cooking: 8 minutes

Servings: 2 chaffles

Ingredients
- 1 tbsp almond flour
- ½ cup mozzarella cheese, shredded
- 1 egg, beaten
- 1 tbsp sweetener
- ½ tsp vanilla extract
- 3-4 chopped mint leaves
- 2 tsp chocolate chips, unsweetened
- A pinch of salt

Directions
1. Heat up your waffle maker.
2. Add all the ingredients to a tiny mixing bowl and combine well.
3. Pour ½ of the batter into your waffle maker and cook for 4 minutes until golden brown. Then cook the remaining batter to make another chaffle.

4. Serve and enjoy!

Almond Chocolate Chaffle and Jam

Preparation: 5 minutes

Cooking: 8 minutes

Servings: 2 chaffles

Ingredients

- 1 egg, beaten
- ½ cup of mozzarella cheese, shredded
- 2 tbsp almond chocolate chips, unsweetened
- 2 tbsp sweetener
- 1 tbsp almond flour
- ¼ tsp baking powder
- 2 tbsp whipped cream for topping
- 2 tbsp raspberries jam, unsweetened for topping

Directions

1. Heat up your waffle maker.
2. Add all the chaffles ingredients to a tiny mixing bowl and mix well.

3. Pour half of the batter into your waffle maker and cook for 4 minutes until golden brown. Repeat now with the rest of the batter to make another chaffle.
4. Let cool for 3 minutes to let chaffles get crispy.
5. Spread each chaffle with raspberries jam and a tbspn of whipped cream.
6. Serve and enjoy!

Caramel & Raspberries Chaffle

Preparation: 5 minutes

Cooking: 8 minutes

Servings: 2 chaffles

Ingredients

For chaffles:

- 1 egg, beaten
- ½ cup mozzarella cheese, grated
- 1 tsp coconut flour
- 1 tsp water
- ¼ tsp baking powder

For topping:

- 2 tbsp keto caramel sauce
- 2 tbsp fresh raspberries
- 2 tsp sweetener

Directions

1. Heat up your waffle maker.

2. Add all the chaffles ingredients to a tiny mixing bowl and combine well.
3. Pour half of the batter into your waffle maker and cook for 4 minutes until brown. Repeat now with the rest of the batter to make another chaffle.
4. Let cool for 3 minutes to let chaffles get crispy.
5. Top the chaffles with caramel sauce and raspberries. Sprinkle with sweetener.
6. Serve and enjoy!

Choco & Coconut Whipped Cream Chaffle

Preparation: 5 minutes

Cooking: 8 minutes

Servings: 2 chaffles

Ingredients

For chaffles:

- 1 tbsp almond flour
- ½ cup mozzarella cheese, shredded
- 1 egg, beaten
- 1 tbsp sweetener
- ½ tsp vanilla extract

For topping:

- 2 tbsp keto coconut whipped cream
- 2 tbsp chocolate chips, unsweetened

Directions

1. Heat up your waffle maker.
2. Add all the ingredients to a tiny mixing bowl and combine well.

3. Pour ½ of the batter into your waffle maker and cook for 4 minutes until golden brown. Cook the remaining batter to make another chaffle.
4. Top the chaffles with keto coconut whipped cream and chocolate chips.
5. Serve with coconut flakes and enjoy!

Cereals & Raspberries Chaffle

Preparation: 5 minutes

Cooking: 8 minutes

Servings: 2 chaffles

Ingredients

- 1 large egg, beaten
- 2 tbsp almond flour
- ½ tsp coconut flour
- 1 tbsp cereals, minced
- ¼ tsp baking powder
- 1 tbsp butter, Melted
- 1 tbsp cream cheese, softened
- ¼ tsp vanilla powder
- 1 tbsp sweetener
- 1 tbsp fresh raspberries, chopped

Directions

1. Heat up your waffle maker.

2. Add all the ingredients to a tiny mixing bowl and stir until well combined.
3. Pour half of the batter into your waffle maker and cook for 4 minutes. Repeat now with the rest of the batter to make another chaffle.
4. Serve with coconut flour and enjoy!

Gourmet Eggnog Chaffle

Preparation: 5 minutes

Cooking: 8 minutes

Servings: 2 chaffles

Ingredients

<u>For chaffles:</u>

- 1 egg, beaten
- 2 tbsp cream cheese, softened
- 2 tsp sweetener
- 2 tbsp coconut flour
- ½ tsp baking powder
- ¼ cup keto eggnog
- A pinch of nutmeg

<u>For topping:</u>

- 2 tbsp keto whipped cream
- 2 tbsp dark chocolate chips, unsweetened

Directions

1. Heat up your waffle maker.

2. Add all the chaffles ingredients to a tiny mixing bowl and stir until well combined.
3. Pour half of the batter into your waffle maker and cook for 4 minutes. Repeat now with the rest of the batter to make another chaffle.
4. Let cool for 3 minutes to let chaffles get crispy.
5. Spread the chaffle with whipped cream and sprinkle with chocolate chips.
6. Serve and enjoy!

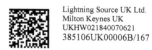
Lightning Source UK Ltd.
Milton Keynes UK
UKHW021840070621
385106UK00006B/167